SGA

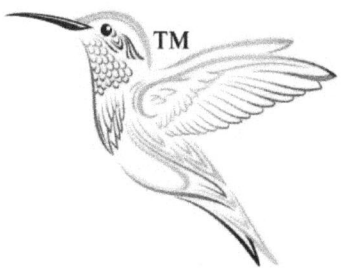

Ian Donald's practical obstetric problems, 7th edition (ID)
Williams obstetrics, 24th edition (W)
Arias' practical guide to high risk pregnancy and delivery, 4th edition (F)
RCOG green top guideline No.31 (R13)
Case discussions in obstetrics & gynecology (P)
<u>15th October 2015</u>

INTRODUCTION

- The proportion of infants with birth weight < 2500 g has increased by more than 20% since 1984, and at the same time, the incidence of birthweight > 4000 g continues to decline.

- LBW = PTB + SGA   LBW = PTB + (FGR + constitutional)

NORMAL FETAL GROWTH

3 phases of fetal growth (W)

Hyperplasia	First 16 weeks	Rapid increase in cell number
Hyperplasia + hypertrophy	Up to 32 weeks	
Hypertrophy	After 32 weeks	Increase in cell size + most fetal fat and glycogen are accumulated

3 factors determining fetal development (W)

- Genetic potential of both parents & is mediated through growth factors such as IGF-I,
- Maternal provision of substrates
- An adequate substrates supply from the placenta & is dependent on uterine and placental vascularity e.g.,
- Glucose:
  - Excessive glycemia (via hyperinsulinemia) produces macrosomia.
  - Reduced maternal glucose levels may result in a LBW. FGR in response to glucose deprivation results only after long-term severe maternal caloric deprivation.
- Lipids: Free or nonesterified fatty acids in maternal plasma may be transferred to the fetus via facilitated diffusion or after liberation of fatty acids from triglycerides by trophoblastic lipases. Lipolytic activity is increased in pregnancy, and fatty acids have been reported to be increased in nonobese women during the third trimester.
  - Excessive transfer of lipids to the fetus results in fetal overgrowth. Overgrown infants have higher placental levels of certain fatty acids, particularly omega-3, and this has been associated with increased trophoblastic lipase expression.
  - Conversely, growth restriction in the third trimester has been associated with decreased maternal lipolysis. This may be related to dysregulation of the triglyceride lipase

gene family, which has been reported in placentas from pregnancies complicated by FGR.

- Amino acids: Amino acids undergo active transport from maternal blood to the fetus, which explains the normally higher fetal concentrations. Amino acids that reach the fetus must first cross the microvillus membrane at the maternal interface, traverse the trophoblastic cell, and finally cross the basal membrane into fetal blood.
  - FGR is associated with lower fetal amino acid levels and higher maternal amino acid concentrations. The etiology of this altered ratio is uncertain.

Hormones implicated in fetal growth (W)

- Insulin and insulin-like growth factors,
- Adipokines; hormones derived from adipose tissue (e.g., leptin; the protein product of the obesity gene, adiponectin, ghrelin, follistatin, resistin, visfatin, vaspin, omentin-1, apelin, and chemerin). Fetal leptin concentrations increase during gestation, and they correlate with birthweight.

Effects of fetal growth

- SFH increases by ~1 cm/week between 14-32 weeks. (ID)
- AG increases by ~1 inch/week after 30 weeks. (ID)

- Fetal growth accelerates from about 5 g/d at 14-15 weeks to 15-20 g/d at 24 weeks, peaks at 30-35 g/d at 34 weeks, after which the growth rate decreases. (W) There may be evolutionary pressure to restrict growth late in pregnancy. Thus, the ability to growth restrict may be adaptive rather than pathological.

Fetal growth versus birth weight (W)

- Birth weight does not define the rate of fetal growth.
- The growth rate of intrinsically SGA newborns approximates that of AGA neonates.

- Diminished growth velocity has been linked to perinatal morbidity and adverse postnatal metabolic changes that are independent of birthweight. Conversely, an excessive fetal-growth velocity, particularly of the AC-which may be correlated with increased hepatic blood flow-is associated with an overgrown neonate.

DEFINITIONS

- **SGA birth is defined as an EFW or AC less than the 10th centile and severe SGA as an EFW or AC less than the 3rd centile (R13).**

- Other definitions are...
  - AC or EFW <3rd or 5th centile (more rigorous, more specific, less sensitive),
  - Mean weights-for-age, with normal limits defined by ±2 SD. This definition would limit SGA infants to 3% of births instead of 10% (W). Thus many at risk fetuses can be missed from surveillance.

- Historically SGA birth has been defined using population centiles. But, the use of centiles customised for maternal characteristics (maternal height, weight, parity and ethnic group) as well as gestational age at delivery and infant sex, identifies small babies at higher risk of morbidity and mortality than those identified by population centiles (R13).

- FGR is not synonymous with SGA. **SGA = constitutionally small & healthy (50-70%) + FGR.** The likelihood of FGR is higher in severe SGA infants. **FGR is a pathological condition in which a fetus has not achieved his genetic growth potential, regardless of fetal size.** As a result, growth restricted fetuses may manifest evidence of fetal compromise (abnormal Doppler studies, reduced liquor volume) (R13). FGR is sometimes defined as SGA with abnormal Doppler indices such as UA PI above the 95th centile or mean Ut PI above the 95th centile (F).

INCIDENCE

- Incidence of SGA (constitutionally small + FGR) is ~10%. (W)
- The incidence of FGR is 4-7% in developed countries & up to 30% in poor resource settings.
- The incidence of LBW (<2.5 kg) [PTB + SGA (constitutionally small + FGR)] in India varies from 15-25%. Of these >50% are due to FGR. (F)

CLASSIFICATION OF SGA (F)

- **Rule out error in pregnancy dating (P):** Pregnancy should be dated according to CRL until 13^{+6} weeks or to HC from 14 weeks.

(P)	Parameter	Error (95%)
History	LMP (excellent history)	14-17 days
	LMP (poor history)	>28 days
	IVF	1 day
	Ovulation induction	3 days
Physical examination	First trimester PV	14 days
	Second trimester fundal height	28 days
	Third trimester fundal height	28 to 36 days
Investigations	CRL 1st trimester **(most accurate)**	5-7 days
	GS 1st trimester	7 days
	BPD (<28 weeks)	5-7 days
	BPD (third trimester)	14-28 days

- SGA fetuses are divided into (R13)...
  - Normal (constitutionally) small,
  - Non-placenta mediated growth restriction, and
  - Placenta mediated growth restriction.

	Constitutionally small fetuses	Non-placental causes (fetal)		Placental causes
		Structural/ Chromosomal	Infection	
Small	From the 2nd trimester	From first early 2nd trimester	Since infected	From the 2nd trimester
Symmetry	Symmetrically small	Symmetrically or asymmetrically small	Asymmetrically small	Asymmetrically small
1st trimester risk for aneuploidy	Low	High	Low	Low
placental hormones (PAPP-A/hCG)	Low or normal	Low	Normal	Low (particularly PAPP-A)
Growth velocity	Maintains	Maintains or reduces	Reduces unless the infection is cured	Reduces Progressively
Feto placental Doppler	Normal	Normal		Abnormal

CLASSIFICATION OF FGR (ID)

Type	Type I (Symmetrical)	Type II (Asymmetrical)	Intermediate (Type I+II)
Time	Early-onset (4-20 weeks)	Late-onset (after 32 weeks)	Intermediate phase
Patho	Active mitosis (hyperplasia) is affected. Decreased number of cells & overall decreased growth potential.	Hypertrophy is affected. Total number of cells is normal but the cell size is reduced. Restriction of substrate supply in utero (uteroplacental insufficiency)	Hyperplasia and hypertrophy both is affected. Decrease of cell number as well as size
Incidence	10-25%	70-80%	5-10%
Causes	Non-placental	Placental	Placental
Diagnosis	All parameters are below 10th percentile for GA	Brain sparing effect leads to normal HC & less AC. Increased flow to brain & heart and ↓sed splanchnic circulation. Liver size is reduced due to ↓sed glycogen stores. (AC decreases)	
PI	Normal	Low (low birth weight & AC)	
Doppler	Normal feto-placental Doppler	Abnormal feto-placental Doppler	
Prognosis	Depends on underlying pathology & the severity of IUGR. Medical interventions are rarely effective as the causative factor is usually uncorrectable.	In case of severe placental insufficiency the head growth curve may also be flattened eventually and the size may drop below the normal growth curve. This may lead to decrease AF, chronic hypoxia and IUFD	

Outdated??? Overlapping seen...

PI (ponderal index) = Birth weight/CRL^3

- Brain sparing in type II allows normal brain and head growth. Accordingly, the ratio of brain weight to liver weight during the last 12 weeks—usually about 3 to 1—may be increased to 5 to 1 or more in severely growth-restricted infants. Because of brain-sparing effects, asymmetrical fetuses were thought to be preferentially protected from the full effects of growth restriction. (W)
- Fetal-growth patterns are much more complex. Study showed that fetuses with aneuploidy typically had disproportionately large head sizes and thus were asymmetrically growth restricted, which was contrary to contemporaneous thinking. Moreover, most preterm infants with growth restriction due to preeclampsia and associated uteroplacental insufficiency were found to have more symmetrical growth impairment—again, a departure from accepted principles. (W)
- Study showed that brain sparing can be detrimental also.

RISK FACTORS/AETIOLOGY

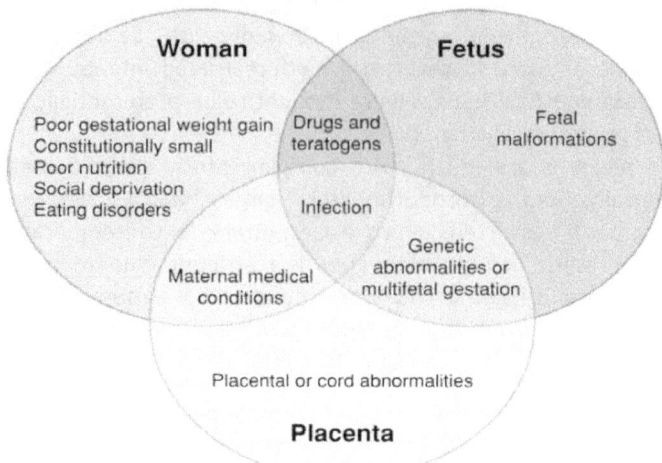

Constitutionally small fetuses

- They are small because they are genetically programmed to be so. Historically, they are considered "symmetrically" small. (F)

Non-placental causes (fetal)

- **Chromosomal abnormality:** In severe SGA, the incidence of chromosomal abnormalities has been reported to be as high as 19%. Among them the most likely are triploidy and trisomy 18. The risk for chromosomal defect is higher if (a) the diagnosis is made before 23-26 weeks' (b) there are associated structural abnormality (c) amniotic fluid volume is normal (d) HC/AC ratio is high or (e) UtA Doppler is normal. (R13) Growth restriction in trisomy 21 is generally mild, by contrast growth is significantly limited in trisomy 18 & 13. Aneuploidic patches in the placenta-confined placental mosaicism-can cause placental insufficiency that may account for many previously unexplained growth-restricted fetuses. (P)

- **Structural abnormality:** All major structural defects involving CNS, CVS, GI, GU & musculoskeletal systems are associated with an increased risk of FGR (e.g., gastroschisis). If FGR + polyhydramnios, the incidence of structural anomaly is increased. (ID)

- **Genetic causes (Inborn errors of metabolism):** Many genes including the gene for glukokinase have been implicated in programming of growth. Certain inborn errors of metabolism like agenesis of pancreas, congenital lipodystrophy, galactosaemia and PKU also causes FGR. (ID)

- **Fetal infection:** Fetal infections are responsible for up to 5% of SGA fetuses. The MC pathogens are CMV, rubella, toxoplasmosis, malaria, tuberculosis and syphilis, although a recent multicentre study found no association between congenital toxoplasmosis and incidence of a SGA. Malaria is a significant cause of preterm birth and LBW worldwide. (R13) Rubella and CMV promote calcifications in the fetus that are associated with cell death, and infection earlier in pregnancy correlates with worse outcomes. Congenital or transplacental tuberculosis is rare, whereas congenital syphilis is more common. Paradoxically, with syphilis, the placenta is almost always larger and heavier due to edema and perivascular inflammation. Congenital syphilis is also strongly linked with preterm birth and thus LBW infants. (W)

Placental causes

- Single umbilical artery, abnormal placental implantation (absence of destruction of the muscle and elastic portion of the spiral arteries in the trophoblast migration), marginal or velamentous umbilical cord insertion, bilobed placenta, extensive infarction, placenta previa, umbilical artery thrombosis, chorioangioma, chronic placental abruption and placental haemangiomas. (ID, W)

- Some uterine malformations have been linked to impaired fetal growth. (W)

- Implantation site disorders (abnormal trophoblastic invasion) may be both a cause and consequence of hypoperfusion at the placental site. These disorders ultimately lead to pregnancy complications such as FGR with or without maternal hypertension. (W)

- Mechanisms leading to abnormal trophoblastic invasion are likely multifactorial, and both vascular and immunological etiologies have been proposed.

- Recently, **ANP converting enzyme**, also known as corrin, has been shown to play a critical role in trophoblastic invasion and remodeling of the uterine spiral arteries. Corrin-deficiency and mutations in the gene for corrin are responsible for abnormal trophoblastic invasion. (W)
- **C4d**, a component of complement that is associated with humoral rejection of transplanted tissues. Study found it to be associated with chronic villitis. Chronic villitis is associated with placental hypoperfusion, fetal acidemia, and FGR and its sequelae. (W)

- **Maternal causes: (R13)**

Major risk factors [OR >2.0] are in bold.

HISTORY AT BOOKING (PRIOR TO 12 WEEKS)	
Maternal Risk Factors	
Age	≥35 years **>40 years**
Ethnicity	African-American & Indian-Asian
Married status	Unmarried
Parity	Nulliparity
Pre-pregnancy weight (BMI)	<20 25-29.9 ≥30
Maternal substance exposure (nicotine & cocaine are vasoconstrictors)	Smoker Smoker (1-10 cigarettes/d) **Smoker (≥11 cigarettes/d)** **Cocaine**
IVF	IVF singleton pregnancy
Exercise	**Daily vigorous exercise**
Diet	Low fruit intake pre-pregnancy
Social	Social deprivation

Previous Pregnancy History	
Previous SGA	Previous SGA baby increases risk to 2 fold, this risk is increased further after 2 SGA
Previous Stillbirth	Previous Stillbirth (6 fold increase), particular those with a H/O previous preterm unexplained stillbirth, due to the association with FGR
Previous pre-eclampsia	Pre-eclampsia
Pregnancy Interval	Pregnancy interval < 6 months Pregnancy interval ≥ 60 months

Termination of pregnancy isn't a risk factor; the evidence regarding recurrent miscarriage is inconsistent.

Maternal Medical History	
SGA	Maternal SGA
Hypertension	Chronic hypertension
Diabetes	Diabetes with vascular disease (R13) Uncontrolled pre-gestational diabetes can cause congenital malformations, risk increases with nephropathy & proliferative retinopathy (W)
Renal disease	Moderate & severe renal impairment (especially when associated with hypertension)
APLS (placental thrombosis)	Antiphospholipid syndrome (two-hit hypothesis)
Congenital heart disease & SLE	Cyanotic heart disease particularly
Paternal Medical History	
SGA	Paternal SGA
Changing paternity	Inconclusive

CURRENT PREGNANCY COMPLICATIONS/DEVELOPMENTS	
Threatened miscarriage	**Heavy bleeding similar to menses**
Down syndrome marker	**PAPP-A < 0.4 MoM (1st trimester screening)**
Ultrasound appearance	**Echogenic bowel**
Violence	Domestic violence
Pre-eclampsia	**Pre-eclampsia**
Pregnancy induced hypertension	Mild **Severe**
Placental abruption	Placental abruption
Unexplained APH	**Unexplained APH**
Weight gain	**Low maternal weight gain (<11 & <7 kg for BMI <30 & ≥30 kg/m² respectively) but it is no longer recommended that women are routinely weighed during pregnancy**
Exposure	Caffeine ≥ 300 mg/day

- **Other causes (W):**
  - Maternal respiratory diseases (cystic fibrosis, bronchiectasis, kyphoscoliosis and asthma)
  - Moderate alcohol intake. It crosses the placenta & act as a cellular poison reducing the fetal growth. It causes fetal alcohol syndrome when consumed in early pregnancy & FGR during 2nd and 3rd trimesters. Consumption >3units/d increases FGR risk 3 fold. (ID)
  - Curtailed maternal blood volume expansion
  - Multiple fetuses
  - Drugs (anticonvulsants, antineoplastic, warfarin, immunosuppressive)
  - High altitude (chronic hypoxia)

In most cases, maternal anemia doesn't cause FGR. **Exceptions include sickle-cell disease & some other inherited anemias.**

Inherited thrombophilias are not a significant factor. (W)

Among the medical disorders contributing to poor intrauterine fetal growth, anemia heads the list. (F)

SCREENING FOR SGA (R13)

- Methods employed in...
  - 1st and 2nd trimester: medical and obstetric history and examination, maternal serum screening and uterine artery Doppler.
  - 2nd and 3rd trimester: Abdominal palpation and measurement of SFH (including customised charts).

History (see maternal causes)

- All women should be assessed at booking for risk factors for a SGA fetus/neonate to identify those who require increased surveillance.
- Women who have...
  - ≥1 major risk factor (OR > 2.0) should be referred for serial ultrasound measurement of fetal size and assessment of wellbeing with umbilical artery Doppler from 26-28 weeks.
  - ≥3 minor risk factors should be referred for uterine artery Doppler at 20-24 weeks.

Biochemical markers used for Down Syndrome screening

- Due to their placental origin, several biochemical markers have been investigated as screening tests for a SGA fetus.
- <0.415 MoM of the first trimester PAPP-A is a major risk factor.
- 2nd trimester DS markers have limited predictive accuracy for SGA.

Uterine artery Doppler

- Role of UtA Doppler in the 1st trimester screening remains under investigation, but in the 2nd trimester represents a valuable tool to assess trophoblastic invasion.

- In high risk populations uterine artery Doppler at 20-24 weeks has a moderate predictive value for a severely SGA neonate.

- Women with an abnormal UtA Doppler at 20-24 weeks (PI > 95th centile) and/or notching should be referred for serial ultrasound measurement of fetal size and assessment of wellbeing with UA Doppler commencing at 26-28 weeks of pregnancy.

- Women with a normal uterine artery Doppler do not require serial measurement of fetal size and serial assessment of wellbeing with umbilical artery Doppler unless they develop specific pregnancy complications, for example antepartum haemorrhage or hypertension. However, they should be offered a scan for fetal size and umbilical artery Doppler during the third trimester.

- The combination of UtA Doppler and maternal serum markers in the 2nd trimester appears to predict adverse outcome related to placental insufficiency more effectively than 1st trimester screening.

- Reference range for UtA PI…(95th centile)
  • 20 to 24 weeks: 1.6 to 1.3

Fetal echogenic bowel

- Serial ultrasound measurement of fetal size and assessment of wellbeing with UA Doppler should be offered.

Clinical examination

- Abdominal palpation has limited accuracy for the prediction of a SGA neonate & severely SGA neonate and thus should not be routinely performed in this context.

- SFH should be measured **(after emptying bladder & lying supine with legs straight)** from the fundus (variable point) to the symphysis pubis (fixed point) with the cm values hidden from the examiner (to avoid observer bias) & should be plotted on a customised chart rather than a population-based chart as this may improve prediction of a SGA neonate. (R13) SFH is measured from upper border of symphysis pubis to the level of uterine fundus. (ID) (P)

- A customised SFH chart is adjusted for maternal characteristics (maternal height, weight, parity and ethnic group). Calculation of customised centiles requires computer software that can be downloaded from the Internet.

- It is simple, safe, inexpensive, and reasonably accurate screening method to detect growth-restricted fetuses. As a screening tool, its principal drawback is imprecision **(sensitivity <35% for detecting excessive or deficient fetal growth & specificity >90%)**. (W) (P)

- SFH is associated with significant intra- and inter-observer variation and serial measurement may improve predictive accuracy. (P)

- Serial measurement of SFH is recommended at each antenatal appointment from 24 weeks of pregnancy as this improves prediction of a SGA neonate.

- Women with a single SFH which plots below the 10th centile or serial measurements which demonstrate slow or static growth by crossing centiles should be referred for ultrasound measurement of fetal size.
- Women in whom measurement of SFH is inaccurate (e.g., BMI >35, large fibroids, hydramnios) should be referred for serial assessment of fetal size using ultrasound.

- Between 18 and 30 weeks', the uterine fundal height in centimeters coincides within 2 weeks of gestational age. Thus, if the measurement is more than 2 to 3 cm from the expected height, inappropriate fetal growth is suspected. (W)

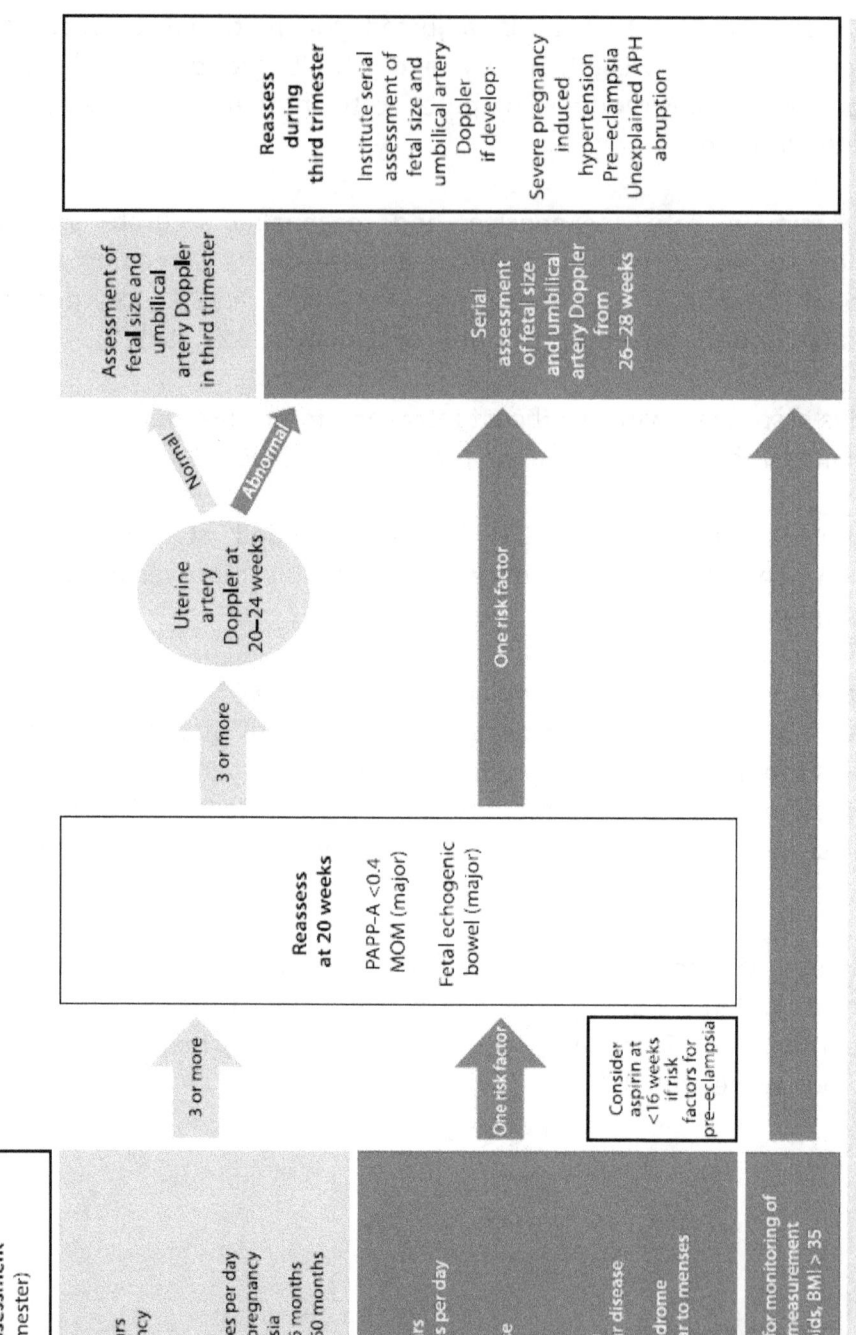

Booking assessment
(first trimester)

Minor risk factors
Maternal age ≥35 years
IVF singleton pregnancy
Nulliparity
BMI <20
BMI 25–34.9
Smoker 1–10 cigarettes per day
Low fruit intake pre-pregnancy
Previous pre-eclampsia
Pregnancy interval <6 months
Pregnancy interval ≥60 months

Major risk factors
Maternal age >40 years
Smoker ≥11 cigarettes per day
Paternal SGA
Cocaine
Daily vigorous exercise
Previous SGA baby
Previous stillbirth
Maternal SGA
Chronic hypertension
Diabetes with vascular disease
Renal impairment
Antiphospholipid syndrome
Heavy bleeding similar to menses
PAPP-A <0.4 MoM

Women unsuitable for monitoring of growth by SFH measurement e.g. Large fibroids, BMI > 35

3 or more

One risk factor

Consider aspirin at <16 weeks if risk factors for pre-eclampsia

Reassess at 20 weeks

PAPP-A <0.4 MOM (major)

Fetal echogenic bowel (major)

3 or more

One risk factor

Uterine artery Doppler at 20–24 weeks

Normal

Abnormal

Assessment of fetal size and umbilical artery Doppler in third trimester

Serial assessment of fetal size and umbilical artery Doppler from 26–28 weeks

Reassess during third trimester

Institute serial assessment of fetal size and umbilical artery Doppler if develop:

Severe pregnancy induced hypertension
Pre-eclampsia
Unexplained APH abruption

Risk assessment must always be individualised (taking into account previous medical and obstetric history and current pregnancy history). Disease progression or institution of medical therapies may increase an individual's risk.

DIAGNOSIS

Fetal biometry

AC & EFW

- Most accurate. (ID) (P)

- AC (transverse section at the level of bifurcation of main portal vein into the right and left branch, the boomerang appearance) has the highest sensitivity and greatest NPV. (ID)

- Fetal AC or EFW <10th centile can be used to diagnose a SGA fetus. (R13) (P)

- Use of a customised fetal weight reference may improve prediction of a SGA neonate and adverse perinatal outcome. In women having serial assessment of fetal size, use of a customised fetal weight reference may improve the prediction of normal perinatal outcome. (R13)

- Routine measurement of fetal AC or EFW in the third trimester does not reduce the incidence of a SGA neonate nor does it improve perinatal outcome. Routine fetal biometry is thus not justified. (R13)

- Change in AC or EFW may improve the prediction of wasting at birth (neonatal morphometric indicators) and adverse perinatal outcome suggestive of FGR. (R13)

- Combining AC or EFW with UA Doppler improves the accuracy of diagnosing FGR. (P)

BPD: It helps to determine the GA & type of IUGR, has low sensitivity as the brain is the last organ to be affected by FGR. It may give false positive results due to alterations in head shape.

HC: It is a better measurement than BPD as it is not subjected to variability as is BPD. The cephalic index (BPD/occipitofrontal diameter) is age-independent and helps in identifying dolicocephaly and brachycephaly.

TCD: Upto 25 weeks, the measurement of TCD in cm equals GA in weeks. Serial measurements have more predictive value than a single measurement.

HC/AC: The normal value of HC/AC decreases linearly from 16 to 40 weeks. An HC/AC >2SD above the mean is predictive of FGR.

FL/AC: FL/AC normal value is 22 ± 2% in the second half of pregnancy & value >23.5% is considered abnormal.

Abnormally elevated HC/AC or FL/AC ratio indicates asymmetrical growth and helps in differentiating a growth restricted fetus from a constitutionally small. (ID)

Placental morphology (ID)

- Grade 0: Late 1st trimester-early 2nd trimester
- Grade I: Mid 2nd trimester to early 3rd trimester (~18-29 wks)
- Grade II: Late 3rd trimester (~30 wks to delivery)
- Grade III: 39 wks to post dates

- Placental changes are not specific for FGR, acceleration of placental maturation may occur with FGR & PIH.

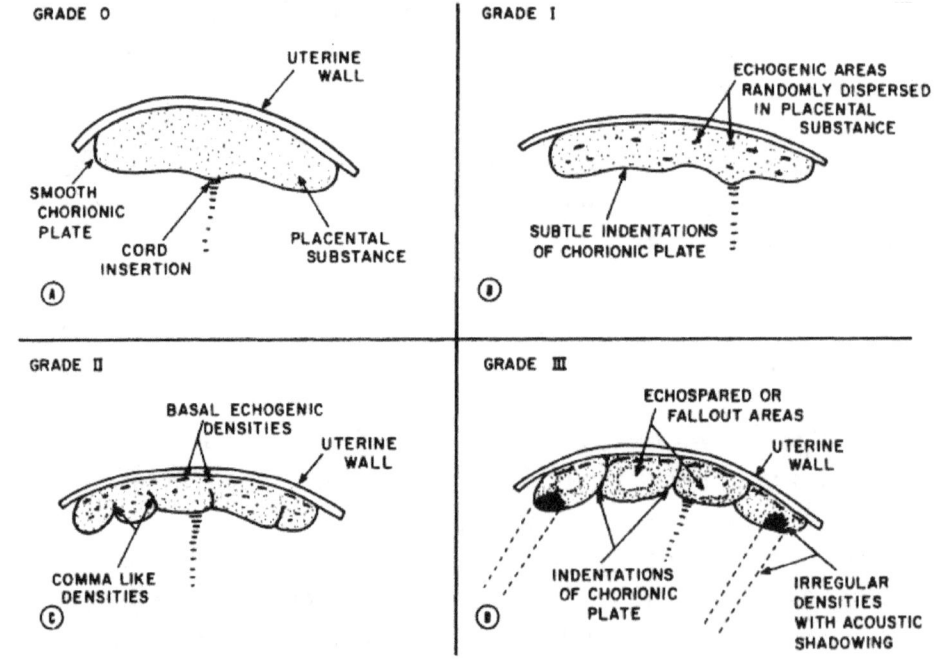

Biophysical tests

- Amniotic fluid volume, CTG and BPP are poor at diagnosing a small or growth restricted fetus. (R13)

Clinical examination

- Clinical examination is a method of screening for fetal size, but is unreliable in detecting SGA. (R13) A lag in SFH of 4 weeks is s/o moderate FGR, while a lag of over 6 weeks suggests severe IUGR. (ID)

Investigations to be undertaken for differential diagnosis

Ultrasound

- Offer referral for a detailed fetal anatomical survey (to rule out structural anomaly) and UtA Doppler by a fetal medicine specialist if severe SGA is identified at the 18-20 week scan. (R13) Fetal echocardiography is done to rule out congenital heart disease.

Invasive prenatal diagnosis

- Karyotyping should be offered in severely SGA fetuses with structural anomalies and in those detected before 23 weeks of gestation, especially if uterine artery Doppler is normal. (R13)

Test for maternal/fetal infection

- Serological screening for CMV and toxoplasmosis infection should be offered in severely SGA. (R13)
- Testing for syphilis and malaria should be considered in high risk populations & who have travelled in endemic areas. (R13)

Other

- Maternal hemoglobin, Hb electrophoresis (hemoglobinopathies), blood sugar (75g 2-hr OGTT), TFT, VDRL (syphilis), renal function test. (ID)
- Specific investigations for APLS should be done in patients with suggestive history and early onset growth restriction. (ID)

Doppler assessment

- UtA Doppler has limited accuracy to predict adverse outcome in SGA fetuses diagnosed during the third trimester. UtA Doppler reflects trophoblastic invasion that is completed at 23-24 weeks. (R13)

- UA Doppler reflects placental function and becomes abnormal if placenta is working ≤50% of its capacity. (F)

- UtA and UA Doppler assessment should be performed at SGA diagnosis in order to detect placental insufficiency and FGR. (F)

Fetal cardiovascular parameters in the evaluation of FGR fetuses (ID)

-    New cardiovascular parameters proposed for evaluation of fetal status...
   • An **abnormal aortic isthmus flow pattern**,
   • **Increased aortic wall thickness**,
   • The **aortic intima-media thickness** is inversely associated with estimated fetal weight,
   • The **myocardial performance index**, a Doppler index of combined systolic and diastolic function, has been shown to be correlated with the presence of cardiac and brain-sparing effects.

FETAL SURVEILLANCE

- The purpose of surveillance is to predict fetal acidaemia thereby allowing timely delivery prior to irreversible end-organ damage and IUFD.

- Where the fetal AC or EFW is < 10th centile or there is evidence of reduced growth velocity, women should be offered serial assessment of fetal size and umbilical artery Doppler. (R13)

Fetal biometry

- Serial assessments of fetal biometry can identify the worsening in growth velocity in SGA fetuses. (F)

- When using two measurements of AC or EFW to estimate growth velocity, **they should be at least 3 weeks apart to minimise false-positive rates** for diagnosing FGR. More frequent measurements of fetal size may be appropriate where birth weight prediction is relevant outside of the context of diagnosing SGA/FGR. (R13)

- **After 30 weeks, mean growth rates for (R13)...**
  - **AC is 10 mm/14 days and**
  - **EFW is 200 g/14 days.**
A change in AC of < 5mm over 14 days is suggestive of FGR.

Uterine artery Doppler (placental development)

- In women with an abnormal UtA Doppler at 20-24 weeks of pregnancy, subsequent normalisation at 26-28 weeks is still associated to a higher risk for SGA compared to women with normal findings since 2nd trimester. The risk for SGA is significantly higher in women with persistent abnormal UtA findings. Despite this, repeating UtA Doppler is therefore of **limited value**. (R13)

Umbilical artery Doppler (placental function)

- In the normal fetus UA Doppler shows presence of diastolic flow by 15 weeks. As the placental resistance decreases with advancing gestation due to trophoblastic invasion, diastolic flow increases. This is manifested as decrease in S/D ratio or PI. Thus the UA shows a waveform with continuous flow during systole and diastole.

- In a high-risk population, the use of UA Doppler has been shown to reduce perinatal morbidity and mortality. UA Doppler should be the **primary surveillance tool in the SGA fetus.** (R13) UA Doppler helps to distinguish constitutionally small fetuses from growth restricted ones. (P)

- High UA PI (>95th centile) with positive end-diastolic flow, AEDF, and REDF reflect that placental insufficiency is ≥50%, ≥70% and ≥90% respectively.

- Repeat UA Doppler...
  - **Every 14 days:** when UA Doppler flow indices are normal
  - **Twice weekly:** when UA Doppler flow indices are abnormal (PI or RI > +2 SDs above mean for GA) with end-diastolic velocities present,
  - **Daily:** when UA Doppler flow indices are abnormal (PI or RI > +2 SDs above mean for GA) with absent/reversed end-diastolic frequencies.

- Although PI has been widely adopted in the UK, an analysis using receiver operator curves found that RI had the best discriminatory ability to predict a range of adverse perinatal outcomes. (R13) PI has the advantage of smaller error and can be numerically analyzed even with absent end diastolic velocity. (P)

- Appropriate reference ranges should be used according to sample site. When comparing repeated measurements longitudinally recordings from fixed sites (i.e., fetal end, placental end, intra-abdominal portion) may be preferable because more reliable.
- Reference range for UA PI at free loop...(95th centile)
  - 24 to 25 weeks: 1.4
  - 26 to 30 weeks: 1.3
  - 31 to 35 weeks: 1.2
  - 36 to 40 weeks: 1.1

Middle cerebral artery Doppler (how the fetus is coping)

- In the normal fetus MCA is characterized by higher impedance to flow as compared to UA and hence it exhibits a low amplitude of diastolic flow in the in the normal circumstances. (P)

- Cerebral vasodilatation, also known as 'brain–sparing effect', is a response of the fetus to chronic hypoxia, and results in increase in diastolic flow and decreases in Doppler indices of the MCA such as the PI. Reduced MCA PI or MCA PI/umbilical artery PI (cerebroplacental ratio) is therefore an early sign of fetal hypoxia in SGA. (R13)

- The 'brain–sparing effect' may develop in 2 scenarios...
  - **In the preterm SGA (<32 weeks) fetus**, where UA was already abnormal, for the worsening of placental circulation. In them **MCA Doppler has limited accuracy** to predict acidaemia and adverse outcome and **should not be used to time delivery.**
  - **In the term SGA (>32 weeks) fetus,** where UA is typically normal because fetal metabolic needs are greater than placental capacity even in absence of placenta insufficiency (i.e., small placenta). In them **an abnormal MCA Doppler** (PI <5th centile) has moderate predictive value for acidosis at birth and should **be used to time delivery**.

- Reference range for MCA PI...(5th centile)
  - 32 to 34 weeks: 1.6
  - 35 to 36 weeks: 1.4
  - 36 to 38 weeks: 1.3

Ductus venosus & umbilical vein Doppler (how the fetus is coping)

- The DV shunts oxygenated blood from the umbilical vein into the IVC, before it joins the portal vein. In the normal fetus, flow in the DV is forward, moving towards the heart during the entire cardiac cycle.

- The DV Doppler flow velocity pattern reflects atrial pressure-volume changes during the cardiac cycle. As FGR worsens **velocity reduces in the**

DV a-wave owing to increased afterload and preload, as well as increased end-diastolic pressure, resulting from the directs effects of hypoxia/acidaemia and increased adrenergic drive. A **retrograde a-wave and pulsatile flow in the umbilical vein** (UV) signifies the onset of overt fetal cardiac compromise. (R13)

- DV Doppler has moderate predictive value for acidaemia and adverse outcome. (R13)

- DV Doppler should be used **for surveillance in the preterm SGA with abnormal UA Doppler** and used **to time delivery.** (R13) DV velocimetry identifies the preterm SGA who are at highest risk of poor outcome at least one week before delivery independent of UA waveform.

- The perinatal mortality in the presence of absent or reversed flow in DV ranges from 63-100% therefore it is recommended that the fetus should be delivered before the development of absent or reversed flow in the DV.

- Reference range for DV PI...(95th centile)
  - 24 to 30 weeks: 0.8
  - 31 to 40 weeks: 0.7
- **Resistive index (RI) = (PSV-EDV) / PSV**
- **Pulsatility index (PI) = (peak systolic velocity - end diastolic velocity) / time averaged velocity = (PSV - EDV) / TAV**
- **S/D ratio = PSV / PDV**

Cardiotocography

- It should not be used as the only form of surveillance. (R13)
- Computerized CTG (cCTG) is (objective and consistent) preferred over conventional CTG (high intra- and inter observer variability).
- Interpretation of the CTG should be based on short term FHR variation from computerized analysis. FHR variation is the most useful predictor of fetal wellbeing in SGA fetuses; a short term variation ≤3 ms (within 24 hours of delivery) has been associated with a higher rate of metabolic acidaemia (54.2% versus 10.5%) and early neonatal death. (R13)

Amniotic fluid volume

- It should not be used as the only form of surveillance.
- Amniotic fluid volume reflects how the fetus has been coping during previous 2-3 weeks. (F)
- Interpretation of amniotic fluid volume should be based on SDVP. (R13) Values ≥2cm are considered normal.

Biophysical profile

- Biophysical profile should not be used for fetal surveillance in preterm SGA fetuses. (R13)
- BPP is time consuming and the incidence of an equivocal result (6/10) is high (15-20%) in severely SGA fetuses, although this rate can be reduced if cCTG is used instead of conventional CTG. (R13) Fetal hypoxemia first affects fetal breathing first followed by AFV, and then FHR variability decreases. Fetal movements and tone are lost with fetal academia, and are late events.

PREVENTION

- Prevention begins before conception, with optimization of maternal medical conditions (e.g., antimalarial prophylaxis for women living in endemic areas and correction of nutritional deficiencies) medications, and nutrition. (W)

- **High green leafy vegetable intake** pre-pregnancy has been reported to be protective. There is no consistent evidence that dietary modification, progesterone or calcium prevent birth of a SGA infant. These interventions should not be used for this indication. (R13)

- **Antiplatelet agents (aspirin)** may be effective in preventing SGA in women at high risk of pre-eclampsia although the effect size is small and should be started at, or before, 16 weeks. (R13) Prophylaxis with low-dose aspirin beginning early in gestation is not recommended because of its poor efficacy to reduce growth restriction. (A13)

- Antihypertensive drug therapy for mild to moderate hypertension in pregnancy does not seem to increase the risk of SGA, but treatment with oral beta-blockers is associated with an increased risk of a SGA. (R13)

- **Smoking cessation** may prevent delivery of a SGA. Women who are able to stop smoking by 15 weeks can reduce the risk back to that of non-smokers. (R13)

- **Antithrombotic therapy** has been used to improve outcome in women considered at risk of placental dysfunction (primarily based on previous history of pre-eclampsia, FGR or stillbirth) and appears to be a promising therapy for preventing delivery of a SGA infant in high-risk women. However there is insufficient evidence, especially concerning serious adverse effects, to recommend its use. (R13)

MANAGEMENT OF SGA/TIMING OF DELIVERY

- At present there is no effective intervention to alter the course of FGR except delivery. Timing delivery is therefore a critical issue in order to balance the risks of prematurity against those of continued intrauterine stay; death and organ damage due to inadequate tissue perfusion. (R13)

- Diagnosis of fetal viral and parasitic infections is important for prognosis and neonatal management. Maternal therapy in toxoplasmosis & malaria may prevent the spread of infection to fetus in utero. (P)

- Women with a SGA fetus between 24^{+0} and 35^{+6} weeks, where delivery is being considered should receive a single course of antenatal **corticosteroids**. (R13)

Preterm SGA

- A proportion of growth restricted fetuses will be delivered prematurely and consequently be at an increased risk of developing cerebral palsy. Maternally administered magnesium sulphate has a neuroprotective effect and reduces the incidence of cerebral palsy amongst preterm infants. Australian guidelines recommend the **magnesium sulphate** when delivery is before 30 weeks. (R13)

- Maternal oxygen administration (55% oxygen at 8L/min): not enough evidence.

- The RCT growth restriction intervention trial (GRIT) compared the effect of delivering early (after completion of a steroid course) with delaying birth for as long as possible (i.e. until the obstetrician was no longer uncertain). (R13) The DIGITAT-Disproportionate Intrauterine Growth Intervention Trial at Term-was designed to study delivery timing of growth-restricted fetuses who were 36 weeks' gestation or older. (W)

- In FGR detected prior to 33 weeks, gestational age was found to be the most significant determinant of total survival until 27 weeks and intact survival until 29 weeks. (R13)

- In the **preterm SGA fetus** with umbilical artery AREDV detected prior to 32 weeks delivery is recommended when **DV Doppler becomes abnormal or UV pulsations appear**, provided the fetus is considered viable (usually when gestational age is ≥ 24 weeks and EFW is > 500 g) and after completion of steroids. Even when **venous Doppler is normal**, delivery is recommended by 32 weeks of gestation and should be considered between 30-32 weeks (given the mortality associated with umbilical artery AREDV alone). (R13)

- Based on available evidence it is not known whether delivery should be recommended as soon as the DV PIV becomes abnormal or whether delivery should be deferred until the DV A-wave becomes absent/reversed. This key question is being addressed in the ongoing trial of umbilical and fetal flow in a European RCT which aims to determine whether delivery based on reduced short term variability on cCTG leads to better neurodevelopmental outcome in surviving infants than delivery based on DV Doppler. (R13)

Term SGA

- If MCA Doppler is abnormal, delivery should be recommended no later than 37 weeks. (R13)

- In the SGA fetus detected after 32 weeks with...
  - An abnormal umbilical artery Doppler, delivery no later than 37 weeks is recommended.
  - A normal umbilical artery Doppler, a senior obstetrician should be involved in determining the timing and mode of birth of these pregnancies. Delivery should be offered at 37 weeks of gestation. (R13)

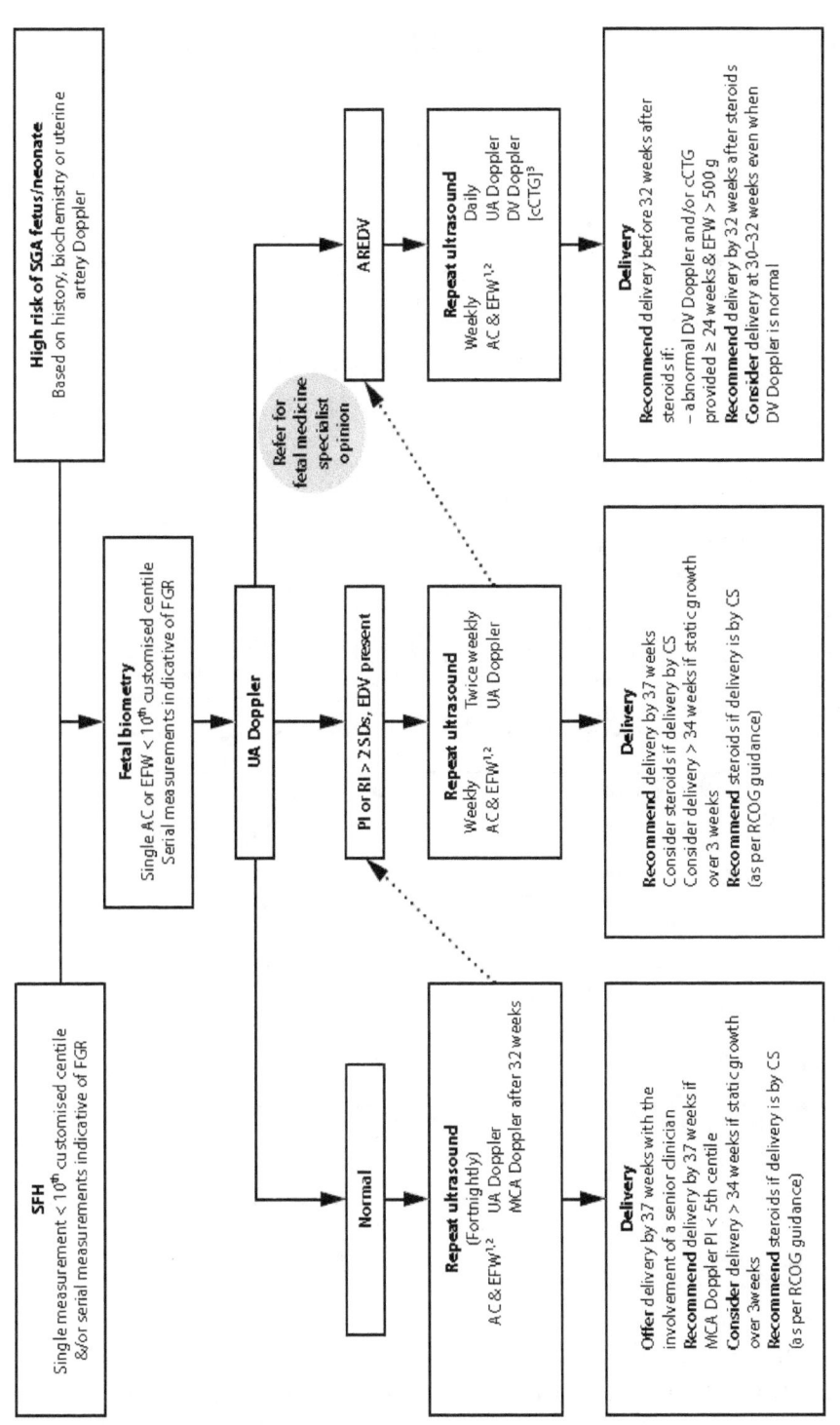

High risk of SGA fetus/neonate
Based on history, biochemistry or uterine artery Doppler

SFH
Single measurement < 10th customised centile &/or serial measurements indicative of FGR

Fetal biometry
Single AC or EFW < 10th customised centile
Serial measurements indicative of FGR

UA Doppler

Normal

PI or RI > 2 SDs, EDV present

AREDV

Refer for fetal medicine specialist opinion

Repeat ultrasound
(Fortnightly)
AC & EFW[1,2]   UA Doppler
MCA Doppler after 32 weeks

Delivery
Offer delivery by 37 weeks with the involvement of a senior clinician
Recommend delivery by 37 weeks if MCA Doppler PI < 5th centile
Consider delivery > 34 weeks if static growth over 3 weeks
Recommend steroids if delivery is by CS (as per RCOG guidance)

Repeat ultrasound
Weekly   Twice weekly
AC & EFW[1,2] UA Doppler

Delivery
Recommend delivery by 37 weeks
Consider steroids if delivery by CS
Consider delivery > 34 weeks if static growth over 3 weeks
Recommend steroids if delivery is by CS (as per RCOG guidance)

Repeat ultrasound
Weekly   Daily
AC & EFW[1,2] UA Doppler
              DV Doppler
              [cCTG][3]

Delivery
Recommend delivery before 32 weeks after steroids if:
– abnormal DV Doppler and/or cCTG provided ≥ 24 weeks & EFW > 500 g
Recommend delivery by 32 weeks after steroids even when DV Doppler is normal
Consider delivery at 30–32 weeks even when DV Doppler is normal

[1] Weekly measurement of fetal size is valuable in predicting birthweight and determining size-for-gestational age
[2] If two AC/EFW measurements are used to estimate growth, they should be at least 3 weeks apart
[3] Use cCTG when DV Doppler is unavailable or results are inconsistent – recommend delivery if STV < 3 ms

Abbreviations: AC, abdominal circumference; EFW, estimated fetal weight; PI, pulsatility index; RI, resistance index; UA, umbilical artery; MCA, middle cerebral artery; DV, ducts venosus; SD, standard deviation; AREDV, Absent/reversed end–diastolic velocities; cCTG, computerised cardiotography; STV, short term variation; SFH, symphysis-fundal height; FGR, fetal growth restriction; EDV, end-diastolic velocities.

MANAGEMENT FLOW CHART ACCORDING TO WILLIAMS 24th EDITION

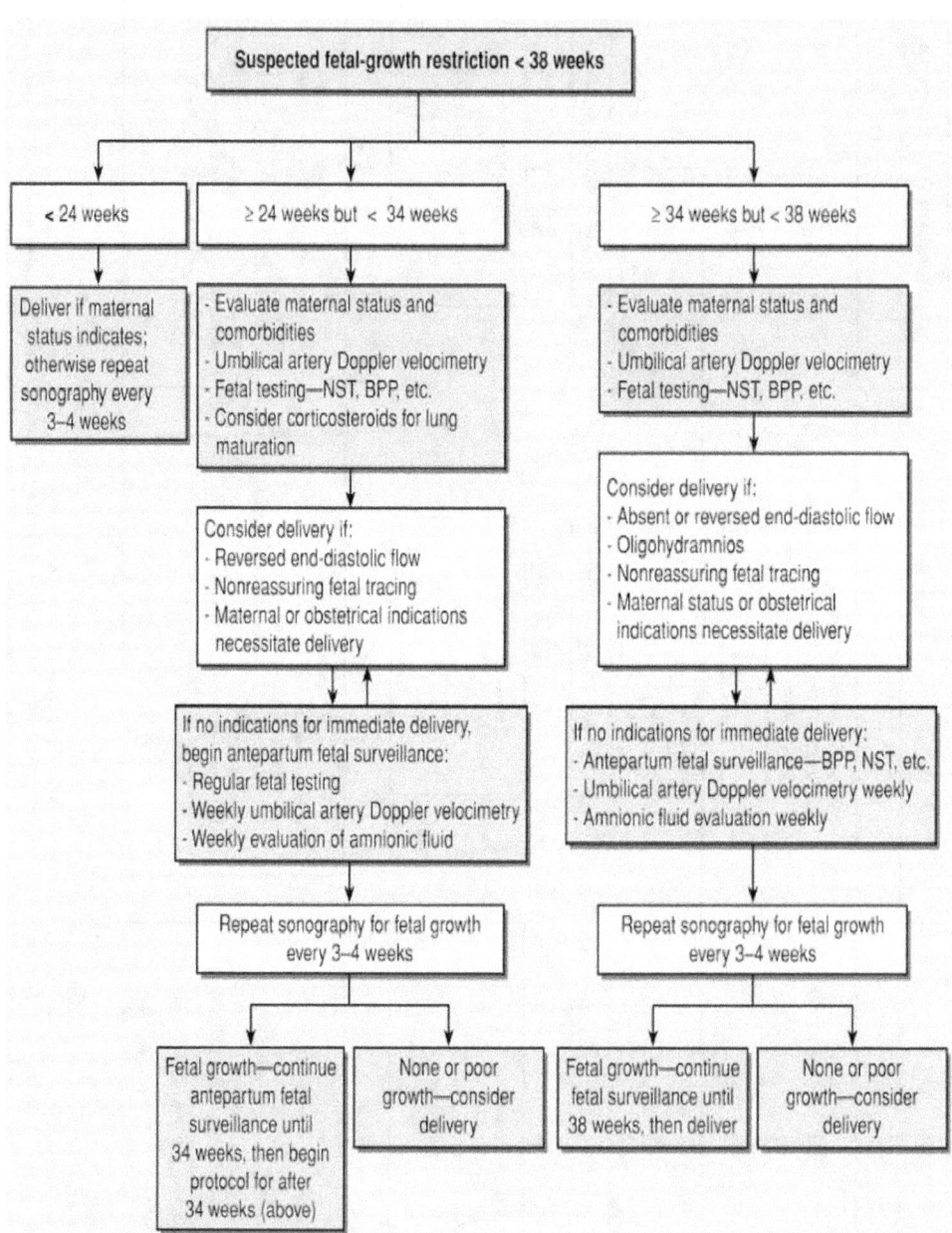

- Management of the near-term fetus: Delivery of a suspected growth-restricted fetus with normal UA Doppler, normal amnionic fluid volume, and reassuring FHR testing can likely be deferred until 38 weeks'. Delivery

is recommended in between 34 and 37 weeks when there are concurrent conditions such as oligohydramnios. (A13)
- Management of the fetus remote from term: As long as there is interval fetal growth and fetal surveillance test results are normal, pregnancy is allowed to continue until fetal lung maturity is reached. (W)

Other management options (ID)

- **Bed rest in left lateral position** to increase uteroplacental blood flow and decrease blood flow to the periphery is not recommended.
- **Maternal nutrient supplementation** (high caloric & protein diets, IV hyperalimentation, consuftion of fish oil, zinc, folate, iron, calcium, vit C & E) is not useful except probably protein energy supplements to poorly nourished women.
- **β_2 mimetics** have no role.

MODE OF DELIVERY

- In the SGA fetus with (R13)...
  - UA AREDV delivery by caesarean section is recommended.
  - Normal umbilical artery Doppler or with abnormal umbilical artery PI but end-diastolic velocities present, IOL can be offered but rates of emergency caesarean section are increased and **continuous FHR monitoring** is recommended from the onset of uterine contractions. (R13)

- Early admission is recommended in women in spontaneous labour with a SGA fetus in order to instigate **continuous FHR monitoring**. (R13) (P)

- FGR is commonly the result of placental insufficiency due to faulty maternal perfusion, reduction of functional placenta, or both. If present, these conditions are likely aggravated by labor. (W)

FETAL & NEONATAL PROBLEMS WITH FGR

Antepartum complications

Fetal hypoxia and acidosis

- Particularly when the growth disturbance is due to placental insufficiency.

Stillbirth

- Fetal death may occur at any time but is more frequent after 35 weeks.

Oligohydramnios

- It is due to decreased fetal urinary output secondary to redistribution of the blood flow with decreased renal perfusion and preferential shunting to the brain.

Intrapartum Complications

- Term and near term SGA fetuses are at increased risk of FHR decelerations in labour, emergency caesarean section for suspected fetal compromise and metabolic acidaemia at delivery. This reflects a lower prelabour pO2 and pH, greater cord compression secondary to oligohydramnios and a greater fall in pH and higher lactate levels when FHR decelerations are present. (R13) (P)

Neonatal Complications

- At birth, the FGR infant is characterized by...
  • Signs of soft tissue wasting,
  • Loose & thin skin and little subcutaneous fat,
  • Scaphoid abdomen,
  • Protuberant ribs,
  • Reduced muscle mass of the arms, buttocks, and thighs,
  • Limp, thin, and frequently meconium-stained umbilical cord,
  • HC larger than the AC.

- BW and in most cases the placental weight are below the 10th percentile,
- Thrombocytopenia and elevated nucleated red blood cell count.

Respiratory distress syndrome

- The main cause of morbidity and mortality in preterm FGR infants.

Complicated pregnancies associated with growth restriction (stressed environment)
↓
Increasing adrenal glucocorticoid secretion
↓
Accelerated fetal lung maturation (?)

OR

Intrauterine hypoxia and ischemia
↓
Leakage of protein (inhibitory surfactant activity) into the alveoli
↓
RDS

Meconium aspiration syndrome

- Passage of meconeum is more common in growth-restricted fetuses, and hypoxia can stimulate respiratory centre leading to aspiration (MAS). Amnioinfusion is only useful in settings where facilities for perinatal surveillance are limited.

Persistent fetal circulation

- Sequel of perinatal hypoxia and acidosis. The pathophysiology is characterized by severe pulmonary vasoconstriction (pulmonary hypertension) with persistent blood flow through the ductus arteriosus. The main signs are hypoxia with mild hypercapnia, right-to-left shunting without evidence of structural heart defect and cardiomegaly. The treatment is adequate ventilation, minimal stimulation, and the use of pulmonary vasodilators (sildenafil).

Intraventricular haemorrhage

- Grade III and IV IVH and PVL are the MC neurological lesions in preterm.

Neonatal encephalopathy

Cerebral edema, intracranial bleeding to infarction

Hypoxic/ischemic brain injury

Seizures, irritability, twitching, and apnea (neonatal encephalopathy)

- It may be followed in some cases by permanent brain injury resulting in cerebral palsy.

Hypoglycemia (<30 mg/dl)

- It is due to...
  • Inadequate glycogen stores,
  • Decreased subcutaneous fat,
  • Deficiency of hepatic gluconeogenic enzymes.
- The symptoms are nonspecific: jitteriness, irritability, drowsiness, apnea, tachypnea, and occasionally seizures. Monitoring of blood glucose levels is necessary in the first 24-48 hours.

Hypocalcemia

- Relative hypoparathyroidism, increased calcitonin level secondary to chronic asphyxia, and increased phosphorus levels resulting from increased tissue catabolism seem to be responsible.
- Symptoms are nearly identical to those of hypoglycemia.

Hyperviscosity syndrome

Chronic hypoxia
↓
Stimulation of the fetal hematopoietic system
↓
Polycythemia (hematocrit >65% or hb% >22g/dl)→Volume overload
(pulmonary edema & CHF)
↓
Hyperviscosity
↓
Slows the blood flow in the microcirculation (pulmonary infarcts and NEC)
Destruction of RBCs (hyperbilirubinemia)

- Treatment involves partial exchange transfusions with plasma.

Hypothermia

- It is due to deficient energy stores and the small size of the subcutaneous fat layer.

Long-term prognosis

- SGA fetuses born at term with or without growth restriction are associated with lower neurodevelopmental scores compared to normal term controls.
- SGA fetuses are at higher risk of developing cerebral palsy.

- Several epidemiologic studies have suggested an association between LBW and the development of chronic hypertension, stroke, dyslipidaemia, cardiac structural changes (systolic & diastolic dysfunction, IHD), structural & functional renal changes (disordered nehrogenesis, renal dysfunction, chronic kidney disease), chronic lung disease, bronchopulmonary dysplasia and type II diabetes in adult life.

CASE PRESENTATION

Presenting a case of Mrs. Ratna Chakrobarty Gravida 2 Parity 1 **(SGA in nulliparous 1.89)**, a Hindu patient of 26 years old **(age ≥35 1.4, age >40 3.2)**, residing at Kadma **(high altitude is risk factor)**, coming from **upper high socio economic class (socio economic status & malnutrition)**, a housewife was admitted in Tata Main Hospital on 12th October 2015 with…

History of 9 months of amenorrhea, appreciating fetal movements well. For elective caesarean.

Origin, duration & progress:

Patient is having 9 months of amenorrhea; admitted for elective caesarean. Patient doesn't have any complaints. H/O fever 15 days back which was low grade, lasted for 1 day, and subsided after taking tab paracetamol.

No history of pain abdomen, bleeding per vaginum, leaking per vaginum.

Obstetric history:

Active married life: 7 years, Non consanguineous marriage.

History of using barrier **contraception** after 1st baby **(H/O using oral contraceptives just prior to conception?)**

Gravida2 Parity1 Abortion0 Living1

> **Gravida1:** Uncomplicated antenatal period. Full term **(gestational age)**, normal vaginal hospital delivery **(mode of delivery)** in 2010. Delivered Male baby of 2.1kg **(previous SGA 3.9)**, 5 years **(interval <6 months or ≥60 months)**, alive and healthy **(history of hypertension, abruption, miscarriages, stillbirth should be ruled out)**.

> **Gravida2:** Present pregnancy, spontaneous conception **(IVF singleton pregnancy is a risk factor)**

>> **1st trimester:** Confirmation of pregnancy done at home with urine pregnancy test, **Prepregnancy weight was 50 kg with BMI 22.2 kg/m^2 (rule out constitutionally small mother)**, booked at Tata Main Hospital, folic acid supplements given, **1st trimester dating scan done**

(using CRL up to 13^{+6} weeks), no H/O fever with or without rash (to rule out TORCH infections, malaria), no H/O exposure to drug or radiation, no H/O bleeding, 1st trimester aneuploidy screening was not done (PAPP-A <0.4), uneventful.

2nd trimester: Quickening at 5th month, oral supplements taken, anomaly scan done (echogenic bowel), 2 doses of tetanus given, antenatal visits at interval of 28 days, weight at the end of 7 completed months was 54 kg (poor or excessive weight gain), no H/O bleeding; pain abdomen; leaking per vaginum (to rule out chronic abruption, placenta previa & PPROM), uneventful.

3rd trimester: Patient was advised ultrasound in view of decreased symphysio fundal height during routine antenatal check up and found to have small for gestational age fetus with less liquor for gestational age on 1st October (35 weeks 3 days). Repeat ultrasound with umbilical artery and middle cerebral artery Doppler was done after 7 days and patient was advised admission for elective caesarean.

Menstrual history:
        Past menstrual period: Interval of 28 days **(regular, any h/o prolonged cycles?)**, lasting for 4-5 days, regular, normal flow, painless.
        Last menstrual period: 26/01/15 **(sure of dates?)**
        Expected date of delivery according to Naegele's formula: 2/11/15 **(EDD cross matched with dating scan)**
        Gestational age: 37 weeks

Past history: No past history of **hypertension, renal disease, asthma, heart disease, diabetes, SLE,** jaundice, **tuberculosis,** blood transfusion, **epilepsy (drugs)** or surgery. **No H/O clots in blood vessels (s/o thrombophilias).**

Family history: No family history of hypertension, diabetes, **genetic disorders or syndromes, hemoglobinopathies,** twins, epilepsy or **tuberculosis.**

Personal history: Patient is having good appetite.
        Patient is taking vegeterian **diet** taking 1 glass of milk with 2 idlis in breakfast; sabji, 2 cup dal and 2 plate of rice in lunch, 1 plate pauha in

supper and 3 roti and sabji in dinner, taking around 2200 kilo calories **(adequate in calories, proteins & micronutrients)**.

Patient is having constipation since 2 days with no complaints in micturition.

No **habbits (caffeine, smoking, cocaine, alcohol).**

No history of any **medication** or **allergy** to any drugs.

General examination:

A pregnant lady, **moderately built, well nourished**, conscious, co-operative & well oriented to time, place & person.

Height 150 cms, weight 57 kg **(weight gain 7 kg)**, **Body mass index of 25.3 kg/m².**

Vitals: Pulse: 90/minute regular with good volume without any radiofemoral delay, Blood pressure: 130/84 mm Hg, afebrile.

No **pallor**, icterus, **edema**, cyanosis, clubbing, **lymph node enlargemen**t. No thyroid enlargement seen.

Breast examination is within normal limits.

Systemic examination:

Respiratory system: Bilateral air entry present, normal vesicular breath sounds present in all lung fields **(rule out respiratory diseases).**

Cardiovascular system: S1, S2 heard, no abnormal sounds present **(rule out cardiac diseases).**

Obstetric examination:

Inspection: Uterus is longitudinally enlarged, umbilicus everted, linea nigra & stria gravidarum present, flanks not full, no scars over abdomen. Hernial orifices were normal.

Palpation [patient should be examined in supine position with legs semi flexed]:

Uterus is 32 to 34 weeks size, relaxed.

Symphysio fundal height is 32 cms, **abdominal circumference** is 35 inches.

Gestational age according to McDonald's rule: $32 \times 8/7 = 36.57$ weeks

1ˢᵗLeopald: On fundal grip, soft, large, irregular, nonballotable mass is felt suggestive of the buttocks.

2ⁿᵈLeopald: On left lateral grip smooth, firm curve is felt suggestive of the back. On right lateral grip irregular, knobs like structures are felt suggestive of the limb of the fetus.

3ʳᵈLeopald/Pawlik's grip: On first pelvic grip firm, regular, curved ballotable part is felt suggestive of head as presenting part.

4ᵗʰLeopald: On second pelvic grip firm, regular, curved mass suggestive of head is felt; hands are converging below the presenting part suggestive of non-engaged head.

Estimated fetal weight according to Johnson's formula: 32 − 12 × 155 = 3100 g ± 275 g

Uterus full of fetus suggestive of oligohydramnios (mention liquor clinically).

No hepatomegaly or splenomegaly (in patients with fever to rule out malaria).

No renal angle tenderness (recurrent upper UTI, chronic pyelonephritis).

A single fetus **(multiple gestation is risk)** is with longitudinal lie, with cephalic presentation

Auscultation: Fetal heart sound is present on left spino umbilical line mid point at rate of 138 beats/min & regular.

Diagnosis: 26 years old, Mrs. Ratna Chakrobarty Gravida 2 Parity 1 with 37 weeks of gestational age with single term small for gestational age fetus with vertex presentation, non-engaged head & fetal heart sound present at left spino umbilical line mid point at 138 beats/min & regular.

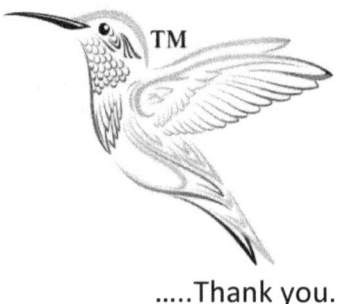

.....Thank you.

www.ingramcontent.com/pod-product-compliance
Lightning Source LLC
Chambersburg PA
CBHW080616180526

45168CB00007B/2938